DECODING DIABETES

NATURAL WAYS TO PREVENT AND REVERSE DIABETES

DR. VISHWANATH

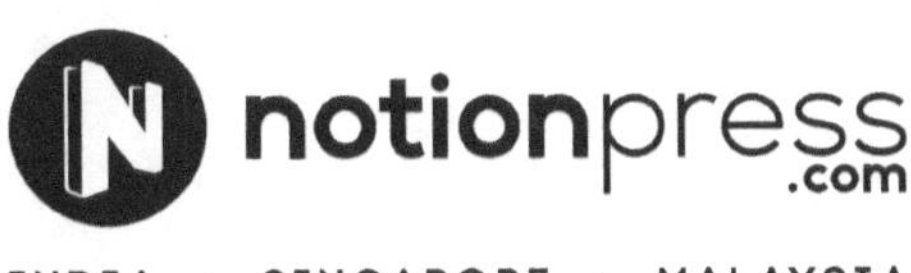

Notion Press

Old No. 38, New No. 6
McNichols Road, Chetpet
Chennai - 600 031

First Published by Notion Press 2019
Copyright © Vishwanath 2019
All Rights Reserved.

ISBN 978-1-64546-638-3

Disclaimer

This book contain opinion and ideas of its author. It is intended to provide helpful and informative material. The reader should consider his or her medical doctor before adopting any suggestions.

Dedication

This work is dedicated to cosmic beloved who inspired me to
write this book.

Immense thanks to my family & friends.

Special thanks to my dear wife Dr. Khushbu Goel &
my son Ishan arya.

Contents

Part – F

Myths and Uncommon Facts on Diabetes

Foreword

Food ranks as the most important among all the basic needs necessary for survival of a human being. During most of the known history of mankind, lack of food acted as the primary limiting factor towards population growth and created social and political systems that we inherit today. One might also speculate that the lack of food was a major contributing factor for the evolution of physiological processes such as lipogenesis (conversion of glucose to fat) and gluconeogenesis (conversion of fat and proteins back to glucose) in animals and human beings.

Since the time of industrial revolution, there has been a gradual reduction in human mortality attributable to lack of food and malnutrition as witnessed by the worldwide increase in human population. This trend accelerated with the arrival of green revolution in the 1960s and one can state with confidence that majority of today's world population enjoys a state of food surplus so that death from famine or malnutrition is mostly non-existent except due to political factors. Curiously, this state has created a strange problem for modern human beings as seen by worldwide increase in the incidence of obesity, adult onset diabetes, and heart disease, the leading cause for which is excessive consumption of dietary calories.

This trend is particularly notable in India where the earlier problem of hunger and famine has been replaced by increased incidence of obesity, adult onset diabetes and heart ailments attributable dietary excess. According to the International Diabetes Federation, more than 72 million people in India suffer from diabetes and the incidence is expected to increase in the coming years. Medical and surgical interventions form the current mainstay of treating diabetes and associated complications. However, given the fact that these ailments were rare during the previous era of famine and malnutrition suggests an alternative treatment approach that primarily relies on dietary intervention rather than medications and surgery.

This book by Dr. Vishwanath is one such effort towards this goal. Though he was trained as a medical doctor to treat these modern ailments by using drugs, he has always maintained a healthy skepticism towards our over reliance on this approach. Particularly notable is his advocacy of intermittent fasting as an alternative lifestyle for healthy living and management of adult onset diabetes. I have personally known Dr. Vishwanath for more than 20 years and he does practice what he preaches including his adherence to intermittent fasting. Dr. Vishwanath convinced me to adopt intermittent fasting as an alternative life style towards healthy living and I can state with confidence that it was one of the best decisions I made in my life. Also, the knowledge I gained during my discussions on this subject with him was helpful in convincing many of my family members to try intermittent fasting as an alternative nondrug approach for managing diabetes. I hope the readers can set aside the prevailing dogma about the role of diet in health and disease and give a serious consideration to many of the actionable advice advocated in this book.

– Sanath Kumar MD
Detroit, MI, USA
March 13, 2019

Part-A

What You Should Know about it and How to Detect It

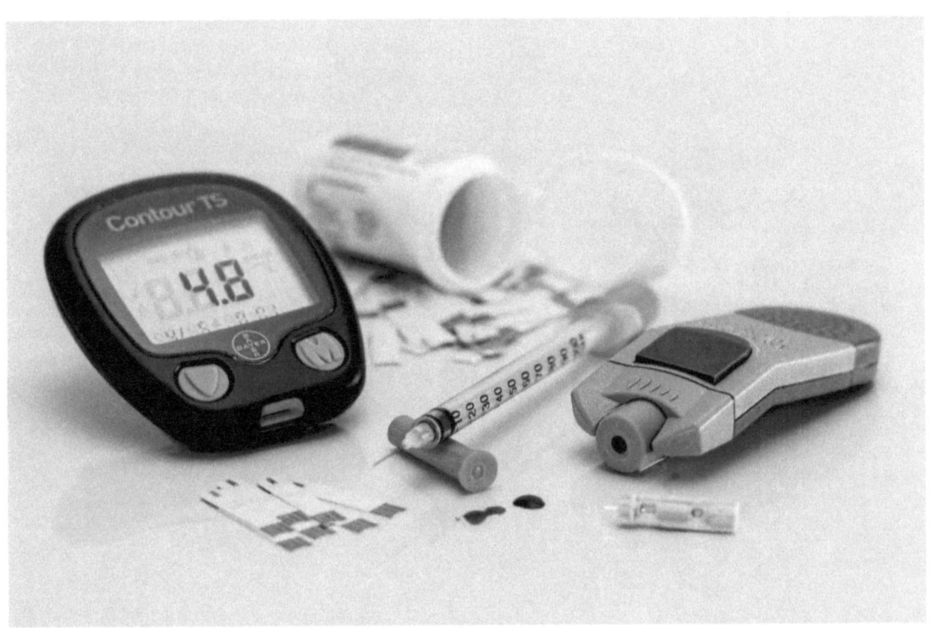

Introduction

Nearly 7 to 10% Indians are suffering from Diabetes.

Many still remain undiagnosed. When I was studying MBBS, Type 2 Diabetes was mostly seen in people above 40 years of age. Today I am regularly coming across people with prediabetes and diabetes in their early 30's in my clinical practices. What is more concerning is how rapidly Diabetes is on a rise consistently since 1980.

GDM – Gestational diabetes for the pregnant woman, is seen in more than 7 to 10% of pregnant women. More than 40% Pregnant women with GDM develop Type 2 Diabetes within 5–10 years of delivery. GDM also puts the next generation to diabetes risk as children whose mothers suffering with GDM tend to develop diabetes when they grow adults. Also people who are in the bracket of pre-diabetes have risen significantly. 10% to 12% of people are in prediabetes stage by age 30 and above. 37% of individuals diagnosed with prediabetes are likely to develop diabetes in four years.

Women have an added risk of developing prediabetes owing to the development of Gestational Diabetes during pregnancy as well as Polycystic ovary syndrome (PCOS).

For the first 5 years after my post graduation, I was happy to treat diabetes with drugs and insulin. Gradually there was a growing feeling in me that I am not doing justice to my diabetes patients as i started realizing I was treating to only lower the high blood sugars and not actually treating the root cause of the disease.

Type 2 Diabetes treatment requires lowering the blood sugars and addressing the root cause which is "Insulin Resistance" through diet intervention and lifestyle changes to reverse the condition.

Many a times there was surging feeling of guilt in me for spending only 15 minutes with diabetic patients as a regular consultation. Actually diabetic consultation demands more time to educate people on diet and lifestyle practices. Type 2 Diabetes is grossly a dietary disease. Counselling every patient on diet and lifestyle by the Doctor is more important than treating with medications and insulin.

Purpose of writing this book is to

1. Prevent people from developing diabetes irrespective of their family history.

2. To make people aware best of diabetic diet practices to reverse diabetes.

3. To make people aware of ancient health practices like fasting in managing diabetes.

4. To make people aware of yogic practices in managing and healing diabetes

5. To educate people about authentic natural remedies and supplements to manage diabetes.

6. To remove myths about diabetes in the minds of people.

To begin with, remove your belief that:

a. Diabetes is a chronic progressive disease.

b. Diabetes is a life time disease and it cannot be reversed.

Type 2 Diabetes is not a chronic progressive disease and most cases can be reversed with proper diet, lifestyle changes and certain yogic practices. Your mindset and lifetyle will play a key role in the process.

*Unless specified the term diabetes in this book means type 2 diabetes.

Chapter 1

Basics of Detecting Diabetes Everyone Must Know

Before we move into the core aspects of Diabetes, let us have a look at what are the various detection methods used. Whatever be the symptoms and signs patients would have, doctors confirm diabetes with the below mentioned tests before starting treatment:

1. Random blood sugar test (RBS)

    A random blood sugar test involves drawing blood at any time, no matter when you last ate. Results equal to or greater than 200 milligrams per deciliter (mg/dL) indicate diabetes.

2. Fasting blood sugar: FBS

    *   It measures the level of your blood sugar after 10 to 12 hours of overnight fasting.

    *   Some times people check their fasting sugar more than 12 hrs of overnight fasting.

    *   It may affect the test results.

    *   It is ideally recommended to check blood sugars with 8 to 10 hrs of overnight fast.

    *   Remember Fasting blood sugars more than 126 is considered diabetic.

    *   Fasting blood sugar between 110 to 125 is considered prediabetic.

3. Post prandial blood sugars: PPBS

    This is the blood sugar level 2 hrs after breakfast.

    2 hrs post breakfast blood sugar levels more than 200 mg/dL is considered diabetic.

    There are also chances of one noticing that the fasting blood sugar level is in diabetic range, but 2 hrs after food, blood sugar show less than fasting blood sugar. This can happen due to reactive hypoglycemia or abnormal high secretion of insulin.

4. Oral Glucose Tolerance Test (GTT)

    The OGTT is suggested as a test when:

    a. Patients having symptoms of diabetes mellitus, but fasting blood sugar value is inconclusive (between 100–126 mg/dl).

    b. During pregnancy to rule out Gestational diabetes.

    You are required to drink a big glass of glucose mixed in water.

    Usually the test uses 75 grams of glucose. The blood is drawn once after 1 hour and again after 2 hours.

    1. If your blood sugar is over 200 mg/dl two hours after you start a glucose tolerance test, you are diagnosed with diabetes.

    2. If it is between 140 mg/dl to 200 mg/dl you will be told you are prediabetic.

Note:

- Gestational diabetes is diagnosed with GTT if 2hr glucose tolerance value is above 140 mg/dl. This arbitrary value is less than guideline value for other individuals.

- Sometimes people will have a normal or high reading at one hour followed by a very low sugar after the second hour of the test. If this happens, it may be due to reactive hypoglycemia.

5. HBA1c test:

    The hemoglobin A1c test tells you your average level of blood sugar over the past 2 to 3 months.

    Guidelines say that one should be diagnosed with diabetes if your A1C reading is 6.5% or higher. It will give an idea about the duration of diabetes onset. If fasting and postprandial blood sugar levels are slightly less than diabetes range (like FBS 120 and PPBS 174) and HBa1c is at diabetic range, then it will clear the confusion in diagnosing diabetes.

Interesting Questions

1. Why fasting blood sugar 125 mg/dL is not diabetic, but 126 m/dL is considered diabetic? Similarly post prandial sugars 199 mg/dL is prediabetic and 200 mg/dL is diabetic, why?

   These numbers are arbitrary. These numbers were set by ADA committee in 1978.

   Initially doctors thought, diabetes complications begin to happen above these blood sugar ranges. Since then various committees, didn't look forward to change the numbers for many reasons including that of maintaining uniformity. Researches and studies have shown diabetes complications can develop even below the diabetes blood sugar range.

2. Is urine tests necessary to diagnose disease?

   No. In the past, urine tests for glucose were used to diagnose and monitor diabetes. Now, they aren't commonly used anymore. Blood glucose tests are more accurate. Urine tests are used to monitor ketone bodies especially in type 1 diabetes and to profile protein leakage when kidneys are affected due to diabetes.

3. How will you know when to test for Diabetes?

   In subsequent chapters I have discussed about the various common and rare symptoms and risk factors which will enable a person to know when he should be considering to take professional advise and diagnosis for diabetes.

Chapter 2

What You Should Know about HBA1C

The hemoglobin A1c blood test reflects average level of blood sugar over the last 2 to 3 months. People who have diabetes need this test to be done regularly once in 3 months to see if their levels are staying within the range. The A1c test is also used to diagnose diabetes.

The recommended cut-off points are

Normal range: 4.5 – 5.6%

Prediabetes range: 5.7 – 6.4%

Diabetic range: ≥ 6.5%

For type 1 and type 2 diabetics who are on treatment the minimum goal is to keep the HbA1c levels under 7%, since keeping levels below 7% has been shown to delay the complications of diabetes. However the higher goal should be to bring it below 6% and subsequently below 5% through a combination of lifestyle changes, dietary interventions and yogic practices explained in the later chapters of this book.

Sometimes the Increase in HbA1c might be the result of certain medical conditions like

1. Kidney failure (uremia).

2. Chronic excessive alcohol intake.

3. Hypertriglyceridemia.

Similarly Medical conditions that may falsely decrease HbA1c include:

1. Acute or chronic blood loss.

2. Sickle cell disease.

3. Thalassemia.

A Note For Pregnant Women:

During the first trimester of pregnancy, the HbA1c target for women with diabetes is 6.1%. During the second and third trimesters of pregnancy, from week 13 onwards, HbA1c should not be used for assessing blood glucose control as it lacks sensitivity and specificity.

What is the controversy on global HbA1c target norms?

The ACP (American college of physicians) targets a Hba1c of 7% to 8%, against the current recommendation of below 6.5% by many other international organisations. This norm of relaxing HBa1c was opposed by many doctors in india. Nevertheless my opinion is HBa1c target of less than 7% is good for Diabetics on treatment. However for an effective long term reversal it need to be brought under 6% first and then 5% subsequently.

However, old age people above 65 years can aim for less stringent control between 7 to 7.5%.

Chapter 3

Are You Prediabetic?

It is also called Borderline diabetes. It's a wake-up call that you're on the path to diabetes. Prediabetes is a condition where the blood sugar levels are higher than normal but not high enough to be Type 2 Diabetes. Prediabetes has prevalence of 10.3% among adults.

The American Diabetes Association classifies anyone with fasting blood sugar between 100–126 mg/DL or the equivalent of HbA1c between 5.7–6.4% as having prediabetes.

Why one should bother about prediabetes?

Prediabetes doesn't have any specific symptoms. If prediabetes is left untreated, there is a very high chance of developing diabetes in next 5 to 10 years. If diet and lifestyle style changes are initiated at the prediabetic stage it can be reversed successfully and will remain that way if sustained as a way of living.

Thus an annual health check to rule out prediabetic is essential irrespective of symptoms after the age of 30.

How frequently to check blood sugar if you are prediabetic?

People with prediabetes, having family history and more than two risk factors like obesity, Polycystic ovarian syndrome must be screened regularly every six months to one year.

Chapter 4

Fasting Insulin Test to Predict the Future Blood Sugar Issues (Pre-pre diabetes test)

Type 2 Diabetes, doesn't develop over the course of days or weeks or even months. It typically starts with a condition called insulin resistance, which can take years and years to show up on standard blood sugar tests.

The Fasting Insulin Test is truly one of the simplest, accurate tests available to detect a trend towards pre-diabetes. It can be called the pre-pre-diabetes test, because it measures your insulin levels, which typically becomes imbalanced long before glucose or HbA1C levels.

Sometimes fasting blood sugar and HBa1c levels may be normal but fasting insulin levels may be high indicating Insulin resistance which is the early precursor to the development of prediabetes and diabetes.

What is optimum insulin levels?

Optimal Fasting Insulin Levels:

Less than 8 (or even better around 5)

Higher levels than 8 definitely indicate some degree of insulin resistance.

Chapter 5

Scary Complications of Diabetes

Knowing about the complications of diabetes is essential to remain aware and make all efforts to prevent them. I see in my clinical practice nearly 30% of people with diabetes suffering from one or other complications.

Here are 4 questions and answers which will help you understand Diabetes complications.

1. What are Diabetes Complications?

    The classic diabetic complications include nerve pain, blindness, and kidney failure. Other complications are heart attacks, strokes, infections, and decreased immunity, gangrene, frozen shoulder etc. Gangrene leading to amputations is the most dreaded complication.

    Doctors call them in less scary names.

    Nerve pain is called "neuropathy." Blindness becomes "retinopathy." Kidney failure becomes "nephropathy." Heart attacks as ischemic heart disease.

2. What causes Diabetic complications?

    All the diabetic complications seem to begin after prolonged exposure to high blood sugars. High blood sugars damages the blood vessels.

    Example: The arteries that supply blood to your heart are damaged by prolonged high blood sugar levels. High blood sugars make these blood vessels stiff and fragile. Over a time they tend to rupture and bleed. When this happens, plaques in heart vessels cause heart attacks.

3. Which complication appears first?

    Usually Nerve damage is the diabetic complication most people experience first. It is caused by damaged blood vessels, in this case the tiny capillaries that supply your nerves are affected.

When nerves don't get enough oxygen they start to die. That is why many diabetics people complain of burning sensations and numbness in their legs.

4. How Long does it take to go into dialysis, blind or losing a foot due to diabetes?

It takes at least a 10 plus years of exposure to high blood sugars to produce full-fledged diabetic complications like kidney failure leading to dialysis, blood vessels damage in eyes leading to blindness or gangrene leading to amputations.

These complications are most likely to happen when your HbA1c has been above 8 to 8.5% for many years.

Hearing all this there is no need to panic. Start working on controlling blood sugar back down to a safer level soon. Most of this damage will heal up, kidney function can improve, nerves will recover and further deterioration may get halted.

I will explain in coming chapters about the best diabetic diet and lifestyle, so that all these complications can be prevented at the early stages. If someone is already suffering from diabetes, suffering can be reduced by diet, lifestyle and tight control of blood sugars.

Part-B

Nutrition and Diabetes

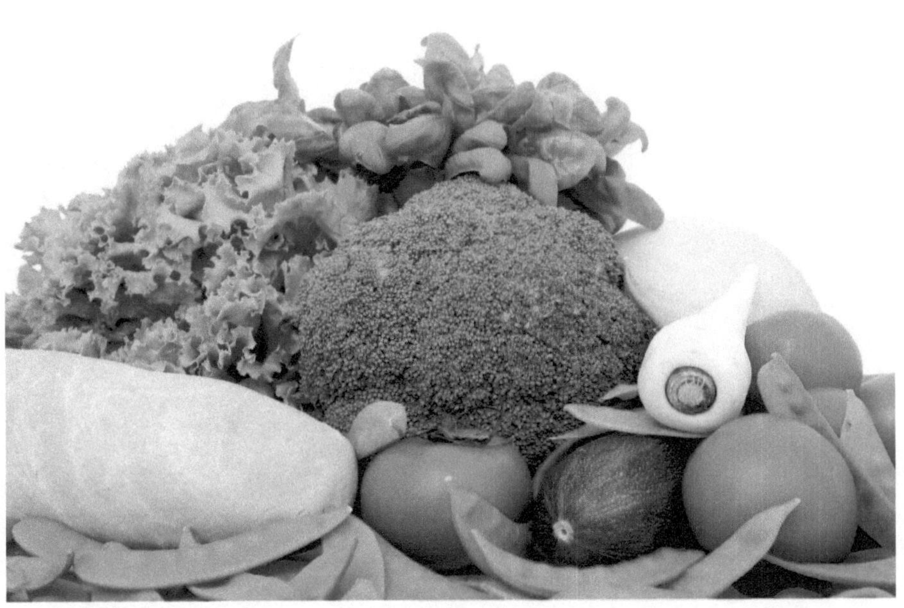

Chapter 1

Breaking Norms & Dietary Misconceptions

If you follow typical "diabetes diet" that many doctors and nutritionists suggest, you may not reverse diabetes, because they are not fundamentally resolving the various internal phenomenons causing diabetes.

Many doctors do not have enough time to explain specifics about diabetes diet. 15 minutes consultation is not enough to explain details about diabetes diet and other aspects that the people must be aware of.

When I enquire about diet during consultation, common answer I get is "we are avoiding rice and eating only wheat chapatis or rotis in meals"

This is completely wrong. Even wheat rises your blood sugars. Glycemic index of wheat flour is almost same as white rice.

The best diet for someone with diabetes is the one that keeps their blood sugars from rising after meals to the levels where diabetic complications occur.

Our food contains three macronutrients carbohydrates, proteins and fats. Carbohydrates increases blood sugars and insulin levels more than proteins and fats. Proteins increases blood sugars mildly. Fats are the least to increase blood sugars and least stimulants of insulin.

Long term Carbohydrates intake stimulate pancreas to secrete more insulin to control blood sugars leading to hyperinsulinemia and insulin resistance which over a period of time causes internal inflammations. Among carbohydrates, refined carbohydrates like Bread, white rice, Maida, wheat, pasta etc are more likely to spike blood sugars and insulin.

So, it's simple.

Best diabetes diet is the one which is low in carbohydrates and with no refined carbohydrates. Presently most people eat 70% to 80% carbohydrates food in their diet. Cut down carbohydrates intake in the diet. To compensate carbohydrates, increase the intake of natural fats and proteins.

People are afraid to eat fat as many health guidelines since 40 years have advised to have "low fat diet." Many studies since last 15 years have proved, that natural fats like almonds, walnuts, olive oil, paneer, coconut and coconut oil, butter, ghee, egg yolk are healthy and does not increase your weight or bad cholesterol.

To conclude, best diabetes diet is **"real food low in carbohydrates, high in natural fats and moderate proteins."**

This is confirmed by many international studies. Nearly 50 patients of mine in 2017–18 nearly reversed their diabetes by following this diet.

In the next chapter, I will explain details about low carb diet.

Chapter 2

Best Diabetic Diets

Do you know when horse gets diabetes, they will be fed "grains free "diet. Actually same diet works best for human diabetes too.

Culturally we are so much used to eating grains. Most of South Indian and north-east Indian diet is rice based and most of North Indian diet is wheat based.

Three types of diets works well for prevention and reversal of diabetes

1. "Grain free-Sugar free diet" with minimal fruits.

2. Keto diet and.

3. Low carbohydrates diet.

These diets help reduce insulin resistance and reverse type 2 diabetes.

What is "Grain free – sugar free diet"?

Around 5000 years ago for nearly 2 million years humans were eating food without grains like rice, wheat, millets (jowar, bajra, bhakri, etc), suji, ragi, oats.

Early humans mostly were eating plant based, animal meats, nuts and seeds for millions of years. They were eating fruits and honey occasionally. Thus by evolution our body is still well adapted to live without grains and sugars.

What to eat in grain free-sugar free diet for Diabetes?

You can eat eggs, vegetables, fish, lean meat, full-fat dairy products like paneer, cheese, vegetables, nuts and seeds. Fruits to be taken in minimal quantity, around 150 grams for 4 days a week is good.

Starchy vegetables like potatoes and corn to be taken in small quantities only.

This will look like an extreme diet for many as we are culturally so much used to grains.

Alternating low carbohydrates diet for 2 months with one month of grain free sugar free diet is better option. There are many evidence backed scientific studies to show the benefits of this diet.

Grain free sugar free (GFSF) diet also has other advantages.

1. It is gluten free to maximum extent.

2. Good for digestive problem.

3. good for weight loss.

4. Good for mental health.

People on diabetes medications must follow this with supervision as sugars may go low with avoidance of grains and sugars.

An Example Diet Plan for grain free-sugar free diet is as below;

Morning:

Coffee or tea without sugar.

Breakfast:

Omelet – 2 to 3 eggs

Paneer Burjee or Tofu Burjee

Green Tea without sugar.

Mid afternoon:

Bowl of mixed fruits 100 to 150 grams. (Low Glycemic Index fruits)

Lunch; 2 pm:

Palak paneer, boiled vegetables with oregano and black pepper,(carrot, broccoli, radish, and little corn)

Tawa roast sweet potato.

Fatty fish or meat for non vegetarians. (Roasted or prepared using coconut oil or olive oil)

5 pm snacks:

Walnuts and almonds (7 to 8 pieces) with pumpkin and flax seeds; (25 grams each)

Dinner at 7 pm:

Same as breakfast or lunch.

You can order 7 days grain free sugar free diet through my website customised according to your health status.

Chapter 3

Keto Diet for Diabetes

Don't confuse Ketosis with Keto acidosis. The former happens with Keto diet, the latter is complication of uncontrolled diabetes.

Ketogenic diet is one of the popular diets since recent years as it aids in rapid weight loss. It is equally good for Diabetes reversal. One issue however is people do not know what can be included under keto diet and what should not be, because of which many people are not on actual keto diet.

In simple terms, Ketogenic diet is high-fat and extremely low-carbohydrates diet, which implies no sugar and no grains like rice, wheat, maize/corn, jowar, ragi etc

This diet shifts metabolism from a glucose-burning machine to a fat-burning one.

Keto diet requires us to consume 65 to 70% as fats, 35% as proteins and less than 10 % as carbohydrates. Remember, in Keto diet you must be ready to consume 70% of food as fats (psychological phobia of fats) and you are not supposed to eat rice, wheat or any other grains.(culturally we are used to eating grain based diets)

Here is sample Keto diet plan:

1. **Breakfast:** paneer bhurji or cheese omelette with vegetables or egg bhurji with coconut or olive oil with vegetables. Coconut chutney can be used daily. (Opt for low sodium cheese while buying from the market)

2. **Snacks at 12 pm:**

   Consume nuts like almonds, walnuts, Macadamia etc.

   Seeds like chia, flaxseed, hemp, pumpkin, sunflower can be taken.

3. **Lunch:** spinach soup with mushrooms and broccoli with boiled Eggs.

Paneer tikka or fried cauliflower

Butter chicken or fatty fried fish for non vegetarians.

4. **Evening snacks:**

Coffee or tea (without sugar) with avocado.

5. **Dinner:** green vegetable salad with cheese/ghee fried paneer.

Eggs in any form

Chicken/fish/mutton for non vegetarians.

What to avoid?

1. AVOID Starchy veggies and legumes, like beans, white potatoes, sweet potatoes, and carrots.

2. Avoid fruits except avocado and berries.

No dry fruits.

3. Avoid alcohol.

After starting Keto diet, it takes 2 to 3 days for ketosis to begin.

Ketosis is a normal metabolic state. Ketones are produced from liver. Don't confuse ketosis with Keto acidosis. Keto acidosis is a dangerous metabolic state that happens with diabetics when there are very high ketones occurring simultaneously with very high blood sugars.

What are the side effects of Keto diet?

Common side effects are

1. bad breath, as the body starts producing ketones.

2. Keto flu' symptoms like fatigue, headache etc.

3. Minor electrolyte imbalances.

Side effects can be minimised with adequate intake of water and salts like Himalayan rock salts. Side effects usually disappear after 1 to 2 weeks of Keto diet.

*Ketogenic diet is a kind of extreme diet.

*Keto diet with Intermittent fasting is highly effective in weight loss, reversing diabetes, reducing high triglycerides and in prevention of neurological diseases like Dementia.

*I recommend Keto diet for short duration of 1 to 2 months with low carbohydrates diet as there are very few long term studies on the benefits of Keto diet.

People with diabetes must follow this diet with supervision as adjustments of diabetes medications and blood sugar monitoring at home is required.

It is not recommended to follow Keto diet for people with kidney disease or any other significant/severe diabetes related complications.

Chapter 4

Low Carb Diet for Diabetes

Low carbohydrate diet is easiest to follow compared to grain free diet and Keto diet. A low-carb diet limits carbohydrates such as grains, starchy vegetables and fruits.

The two fundamental principles of a Healthy Diet and one that will help in your attempt to Diabetes control and reversal is:

1. Eat food as natural as possible.

2. Have a diet low in Carbohydrate with moderate protein and moderately high in natural healthy fats (LCHF Diet).

Low carbohydrate Diet means diet which contains less than 25% as carbohydrates.

30 to 40% as proteins and

40 to 50% healthy natural fats.

Here is a list of foods to be included in low carbohydrates diet.

Vegetables:

Broccoli, Cauliflower, Tomatoes, spinach, Cucumber, capsicum Drumstick, Radish, etc.

sweet potato as an alternative to potato

Make nearly 50% of your diet with vegetables.

Staple:

Millets such as Foxtail (Navane), Barnyard (Oodalu), Araka (Kodo), Little (Samai) and Brown Top (Korale) and ragi.

Replace your White Rice and wheat with red rice, brown rice, black rice, Quinoa, and Oats,

Fruits and dry fruits:

Apple, Avocado, Guava, All Berries, Grapes, Kiwi, Pomegranate, Lemon and Amla.

Today's hybrid fruits are more sugary. Eat fruits in moderation.

Eat a mix of any two fruits: not more than 150 gms per day

Dry fruits like raisins not more than 50 gms. One cup of raisins have over 80 grams of sugar while a cup of grapes have about 15 grams or less.

Nuts and seeds:

Walnuts, Almonds, Pista, Chestnut, Peanuts, Pumpkin seeds, chia seeds and flax seeds.

Daily eat any two nuts or any two seeds in moderation. Horse Gram is a pulse that you can add to your diet, it very effective. Under the blog section in my website www.drvishwanath.com you will find details about all these and much more. Every week the blog is updated with various helpful health topics and methods for people to understand, follow and take benefit of. After reading this book, it would make sense to visit the blogs too.

NON vegetarian food:

Eggs, Organically Grown Chicken, Lean Meats, Fish.

Must Include Spices:

Turmeric, Cinnamon, Jeera, Ginger and Dry Ginger, Garlic,

Oils for cooking:

Virgin Coconut Oil, Virgin Olive Oil, Sesame oil and cold pressed groundnut oil.

DO's

1. Eat adequate protein with each meal. Proteins reduce cravings and regulate blood sugars.

    Example of vegetarian proteins are Horse Gram, Dals, Channa, Soya, Yogurt, Broccoli, Paneer, Tofu etc…

    Eggs and fish are recommended protein sources for non vegetarians.

2. Eat Natural fats like egg yolk, olive oil, coconut, avocado, paneer, almonds, walnuts, home made ghee and butter in small quantity.

Natural fats are healthy.

DONOTs

1. No White Rice, No wheat, No Rawa, No Maida, No white breads and No sugar in any form.

2. No White Sugar or Brown Sugar.

3. No Sweets and Desserts. (Only Once or twice in a month as a cheat shot in small quantity)

4. Avoid Refined Food, Processed Food and Packaged foods.

There are enough case studies and examples showing better diabetes control with low carbohydrates diet. In my clinical practices too i have seen good results with this diet.

You can get the 7 day low carbohydrate diet plan customised to your health status in the Programs and Therapies page of my website.

Chapter 5

Fruits and Diabetes

This chapter dwells on two important questions related to fruit consumption.

WHAT ARE THE BEST FRUITS FOR DIABETICS?

HOW MUCH FRUIT IS ENOUGH FOR DIABETICS?

Fruit can be part of a diabetes-friendly diet. They are loaded with essential vitamins, minerals, fiber, and antioxidants. They taste good and are refreshing, filling, and also add color to your plate.

The key to selecting the right fruit is to choose the right kinds and appropriate portions. As they can contain high amounts of carbohydrates that can affect your blood sugar levels, you need to eat moderate quantity of fruits.

Here are 5 Tips to Enjoy Fruits If You Are a Diabetic

Eating fruits is healthy but eating in moderation is better.

1. Always eat fruits that are fresh, local and in season. Raw fruits are best as it contains fibers and retains most of the essential nutrients.

2. Never consume fruit juice as it's devoid of all the fiber and contains added sugars which would spike blood sugar levels.

3. Fruits should not be eaten with your main meals, its best to have fruits in between meals and as a snack. This is because fruits act as fillers in the diet, as they are rich in fibers.

4. Eat fruits with some nuts to balance the glycemic load. A low glycemic load will indicate low level of sugar in blood.

5. Sprinkle fruits with grounded cinnamon powder which is very helpful in balancing blood sugar levels. As cinnamon has good blood sugar lowering properties.

6. Always eat fruit in moderation. Fruit is nature's candy. They provide natural sugars which can be easily digested.

I personally recommend eating 100 gm fruit per day – 4 to 5 days in a week.

What Are The Diabetic Friendly Fruits You Can Have?

Here I am listing the 15 best fruits that can be taken by diabetics as a part of their regular diet.

1. Strawberries

    There are 15 g of carbohydrate in 1 bowl of Strawberries. One bowl of strawberries contains almost as much vitamin C as one cup of orange juice. It also contains folic acid. In addition, strawberries are rich in potassium and are packed with antioxidants, such as anthocyanins, and quercetin. Making it an all-round low-calorie choice for diabetics.

2. Apple

    Apples contain vitamin C, fiber and several antioxidants. A medium sized apple contains 95 calories, 25 grams of carbohydrates and 14% of the daily value for vitamin C. You can find most of the nutrients in apple's skin. Also, apples contain large amounts of water and fiber, which is the reason you feel full after taking an apple. The fibers present in apple keeps the sugar levels in check.

3. Water Melon

    Watermelon contains high amounts of fiber and moderate amounts of lycopene. This is the pigment that gives the fruit its color. It's also a powerful antioxidant. It is suggested that lycopene is involved in reducing cardiovascular diseases. It has been observed that diabetics suffer from cardiovascular diseases at some point of time, so a moderate amount of this fruit can provide good benefits.

4. Papaya

    Papaya is a great choice for diabetics as it is loaded with natural antioxidants. Diabetics are susceptible to many complications, including heart and nerve damage resulting from irregular blood sugar levels.

5. Orange

    Orange is a rich source of flavonoids and phenolic acid, which have shown tremendous protective abilities, especially in case of diabetics. Citrus fruits are excellent when it comes to breaking down glucose, as they not only delay glucose update but also inhibit the movement or transport of glucose through the intestines and liver.

6. Mosambi

    Mosambi juice with amla and honey on empty stomach is very beneficial for diabetic patients.

7. Guava

    Guavas are rich in fiber that helps ease constipation, a common concern among diabetic patients' community, in addition to that it can also lower the chances of developing type-2 diabetes as fibers keep the sugar levels in control.

8. Pomegranate

    Pomegranate is a super fruit as it contains the richest combinations of antioxidants of all fruits in the fruit kingdom that can protect you from free-radicals and chronic diseases. So it can be incorporated in the daily diet for multiple health benefits.

9. Grapes

    Grapes contain Resveratrol, which is also found in some berries, it has the property of modulating the blood glucose response by affecting how the body secretes and uses insulin available in the bloodstream. Hence grapes can be a good choice keeping its nutritional benefits in mind.

10. Blueberries

    There are 15 grams of carbohydrate in 3/4 cup. Blueberries are the berry with the most antioxidants and contain flavonoids and resveratrol which is a polyphenolic compound naturally found in peanut, grapes, red wine, and some berries.

11. Mangoes

Mangoes are regarded as the king of fruits, a ripe mango can contain up to 31 grams of sugar, but its glycemic load is only 10. The fiber in mango helps in limiting the rapid absorption of the sugars. Thus keeping balanced sugar level. It is advised to eat mango in moderation.

12. Pears

Pears are an excellent source of fiber and also vitamin K, which makes them a great addition to any diabetes diet plan.

13. Jamun

Jamun improves blood sugar control. It is 82% water and 14.5% carbohydrates. The best thing about Jamun is that it has a hypoglycemic effect that helps in reducing blood and urine sugar levels. In addition to the pulp, the seed of Jamun are also very beneficial in controlling diabetes.

14. Jackfruit

Picture Source: Epicurious

Jackfruit contains many essential nutrients such as Vitamin A, C, niacin, manganese, magnesium, and calcium etc, a great option for diabetics. It also improves insulin resistance in diabetic people. Raw jackfruit has a lower glycemic index.

Learn more about the health benefits of Jackfruit. Check out my blog on the same topic –Surprising Health Benefits of Jackfruit That You Must Know!

15. Cherries

Tart Cherries are great for diabetic people as their GI (Glycemic Index) value is 20 and in some cases, less than 20.

A diabetic should never stop eating fruits; in fact they should make it a part of their daily diet. Only the quantity of serving should be in moderation as fruits play a key role in detoxification.

Chapter 6

Can Diabetics Take Alcohol?

Research shows that a moderate amount of alcohol will not have a serious effect on the blood sugar levels of people with type 1 or 2 diabetes. However, It is necessary to know how alcohol impacts diabetes.

A. Alcohol Can Increase or Decrease Blood Sugar.

Alcohol affects individuals depending on age, gender and body weight. Moderate alcohol intake can increase blood sugars and heavy intake will cause low sugar (Hypoglycaemia).

Alcohol inhibits the liver's ability to release glucose into the bloodstream and can cause a low blood sugar attack. Liver gives preference to detoxifying the alcohol over metabolising the food we consume

B. Alcohol Interferes with Action Of Diabetic Medications.

Diabetes drug sulfonylureas and insulin can cause hypoglycemia by interacting with alcohol.

Another drug metformin in higher doses can cause lactic acidosis with heavy alcohol consumption.

C. Alcohol Increases Your Appetite Making You To Eat More.

Alcohol increases the craving for the food which affects blood sugars. Many times, it is not the alcohol which does harm to health, it is the junk foods eaten with alcohol hat does

D. Alcohol Increases Triglycerides and Alcohol Can Also Cause Weight Gain.

How much is not Too Much?

Most people with diabetes can safely drink alcohol in moderation and here is a small info about how much alcohol can be consumed while you are a Diabetic, if you cannot stay away from the saying CHEERS!!!

a. 150 to 200 ml of Wine.

b. 2 pints of Regular Beer.

c. 2 to 3 small pegs (30ml) of hot drinks like Gin, Vodka or Whisky.

d. Never try patiala pegs (90ml).

TIPS FOR DIABETICS TO DRINK ALCOHOL SAFELY

1. Do not drink on an empty stomach.

2. Don't Drink when your blood glucose level is low or high.

3. Do not replace food with alcohol.

4. Drink with a zero-sugar and zero-alcohol drink (water, soda).

5. Hydrate well: Keep sipping water to avoid dehydration.

6. Monitor your blood sugars before and after drinking.

7. Avoid drinks if you have coexisting liver or kidney problems.

So I hope with these, one can be in control of and manage alcohol consumption accordingly.

Chapter 7

Vitamins Essential for Diabetics

Before we begin, here is a Note on Vitamin Supplements for Diabetics.

Vitamin Supplements may help you get adequate amounts of important nutrients in case your food is unable to provide these, but these supplements cannot replace a good nutrient diet. Vitamin supplements contain active ingredients and these may have some side-effects. It is best to get these vitamins in diet in its natural form rather than getting it through capsules or tablets.

There are 13 vitamins needed for human body. Below mentioned 6 vitamins are required for diabetics as they help in bettering body's ability to use INSULIN, thus keeping your blood sugar under control. They also help in preventing and managing diabetes complications.

1. Vitamin B6(pyridoxine)

2. Vitamin B12

3. BIOTIN (vitamin B7)

4. Vitamin C

5. Vitamin D

6. Vitamin E

1. VITAMIN B6:

It prevents glycation which is responsible for diabetes complications. It also supports nerve health which is helpful in preventing diabetic neuropathy. Foods high in vitamin B6 include bananas, spinach, broccoli, red capsicum, baked potatoes and chickpeas. Pista is also a good source.

Lean chicken, meat and fish are good non-veg sources.

2. VITAMIN B12:

Vitamin B12 deficiency can occur in diabetics who take medication Metformin. Vitamin b12 is very essential for diabetes neuropathy management.

Note: Along with Vitamin B12 and B6, Vitamin B1 also helps in controlling Diabetes Neuropathy (nerve damage).

Vegetarians are at risk of vitamin B12 deficiency. It is mostly found in non-vegetarian food.

Veg sources: Milk, yogurt, Butter milk and fortified soy milk.

Non-veg sources; liver and kidney meat, seafood and Egg yolks.

3. BIOTIN:

It works in synergy with insulin. It increases the activity of glucokinase enzyme which is responsible for glucose utilisation.

Food sources: Egg yolk, Almonds, Cauliflower, Mushrooms, Sweet Potatoes and Salmon.

4. VITAMIN D:

Vitamin D deficiency alters insulin synthesis and secretion thereby negatively impacting blood sugars.

You can increase your intake through foods such as fatty fish, mushrooms, cheese, soya products Sunflower seeds and egg yolk which are good sources.

Sunlight is the best natural source. So a morning walk would be a good idea. Vitamin D supplement is must now a days as many are deficient.

5. VITAMIN C:

It is very essential vitamin for Diabetics. Type 1 diabetics generally have low vitamin C levels. By increasing the amount of vitamin C, the amount of sorbitol may be lowered.

Sorbitol is a harmful sugar when it accumulates, leads to increased risk of diabetic complications. In the case of type 2 diabetics, vitamin C may play a role in improving glucose tolerance and preventing oxidative damage. It is also good for arterial health.

Food sources; Citrus fruits, Amla, Leafy green vegetables such as spinach capsicum (yellow), broccoli, and green chillies. Strawberries, Papaya and Guava in fruits.

6. VITAMIN E:

Vitamin E can oxygenate the blood, and improve the activity of insulin within the body. It prevents Diabetes complications with its antioxidant properties.

Almonds, peanuts, hazel nuts, avocado and sunflower seeds are all high in vitamin E. So are spinach and broccoli.

All the essential vitamins for Diabetes must be taken in natural forms. If not possible, vitamin supplements can be considered.

My Personal Recommendation Is

A. **Make 50% Of Your Diet As Vegetables (Eat Multiple Multicolored Vegetables).**

B. **Daily Eat Any Two Nuts Among Almonds, Walnuts, Hazelnuts And Peanuts In Small Quantity.**

C. **Daily Eat Any Two Seeds Like Chia, Pumpkin, Flaxseed, Methi And Sunflower.**

D. **Daily Eat 100 To 150 Gm Mix Of Any 3 Fruits. One Among Them Must Be Citrous Fruit.(Vitamin C)**

E. **Use Multiple Grains For Roti Instead Of Using Only Wheat.**

F. **Eat 2 Or 3 Eggs Daily.**

G. **Fish Twice A Week For Non Vegetarians.**

With The Above Recommendation, Most Of The Vitamins Are Included In Diet. Taking too many supplements is not a good option as Diabetic people are already on multiple medications and it may lead to side effects. Do remember supplements are not medicines, so one cannot really replace the medicine with supplements.

6 Crucial Nutrients Needed for All Diabetics

These Elements helps in blood sugar control as they are indirectly involved in glucose metabolism and insulin action. Knowledge about these nutrients will make you understand the importance of balanced diet.

1. Alpha lipoid acid

2. Chromium

3. Inositol

4. Magnesium

5. Coenzyme 10

6. Zinc

1. ALPHA LIPOIC ACID: It is an antioxidant which helps in:

    - Improving insulin sensitivity

    - Lowering blood sugar

    - Improving blood vessel tone, and

    - Decreasing inflammation.

Natural sources: Spinach, Broccoli, Peas and Tomatoes.

Moreover, dietary ALA has limited benefit to the body as it is bound to an amino acid (lysine) and cannot freely circulate to perform its function.

Recommended Dose is 600 mg per day.

2. CHROMIUM:

Chromium protects the receptors and allows effective binding of insulin, thereby increasing insulin sensitivity. Exercise increases the concentration of tissue chromium. Chromium may have a role to play in pre-diabetics and women suffering from gestational diabetes.

Natural sources of chromium are sea foods, Brown rice, Broccoli and mushrooms. It Is better to increase chromium intake through food.

3. INOSITOL:

There is conclusive evidence of the efficiency of D-Chiro inositol and Myo inositol in increasing insulin sensitivity and helping bring down blood glucose levels. But inositol does have a potential to be used for Gestational diabetes.

Myo-inositol is most effective in issues concerning female health like fertility and PCOD.

Inositol may have a role to play in reversing the effects of diabetic neuropathy (nervous damage) caused by diabetes.

Inositol rich foods are eggs and meat.

Citrous fruits like oranges, peaches and pears are good sources.

Recommended dose is 600 mg per day. (is this for supplements)

4. CO ENZYME 10:

Co enzyme 10 produces energy as well as act as antioxidant. Many diabetic people take cholesterol lowering drugs called statins. Statins brings down the level of coenzyme 10. Statins impair insulin secretion as well as reduce the sensitivity of fat cells to insulin, leading to diabetes.

Anti-diabetes medications including Acetohexamide, Chlorpropamide, Glipizide, Glyburide, Tolazamide. Tolbutamide reduces coenzyme 10. Supplementing with the right amount of CoQ10 can help in dealing with statin-induced diabetes.

For most people, 200 mg a day of CoQ10 supplementation works. Getting through food sources is not adequate.

5. MAGNESIUM:

Magnesium improves the functioning of cells in pancreas thereby helping in prevention of diabetes.

Magnesium improves insulin sensitivity, it relaxes muscles so insulin resistance is reduced, it is also helpful in diabetes Neuropathy. It helps in conversion of glucose to glycogen.

Magnesium rich foods are green leafy vegetables, Almonds, pumpkin seeds, mackerel fish, avocado and dry fruits like fig and apricots.

Magnesium citrate is a safe supplement. However It is not required as it is possible to get enough magnesium through foods naturally.

6. ZINC:

Zinc is a crucial element in insulin metabolism. Zinc may also act to protect beta cells of pancreas from destruction. Zinc reduces hyperinsulinemia in PCOD patients.

Type 1 diabetics are often zinc deficient, and intake of zinc have been shown to lower blood sugar levels in some type 1 cases.

pumpkin seeds, chickpeas, spinach and cashews are zinc rich foods. Meat and poultry are also good sources.

Final Remarks

These essential elements and minerals are not the replacement to diabetes medications.

It's regular supplementation through diet helps in better blood sugar control. Those which are not adequately available through foods can be taken in the form of tablets or capsules. Supplements are to be taken with the advice of physician or diabetologist.

Chapter 9

Natural Remedies and Supplements for Diabetes

These natural supplements mentioned below also help in preventing the risk of type 2 diabetes and in maintaining blood sugar levels. Though there is limited scientific evidence for many natural supplements, they are time tested across centuries especially in India and some find extensive use in Ayurveda.

NATURAL HERBS, FRUITS AND SPICES.

- Ashwagandha

- Cinnamon

- Gymnesia extract

- Berberine (Daruhaldi)

- Pomegranate Extract

- Noni fruit

- Jamun fruit and seeds

- Okra (Bhindee)

- Horse Gram – The Miracle Pulse.

- Aloe vera

- Bitter gourd

- Fenugreek

- Ginger

- Garlic

- Saffron

- Cloves

- Amla

- Turmeric

- Green tea extract

- Fish oil

- Apple cider vinegar.

Include few of them in your daily diet small quantities and it can work wonders when it becomes a regular inclusion. You can visit my blogs at www.drvishwanath.com to access more details of the above listed herbs, fruits and spices.

Few of them like ashwagandha, Gymnesia and Berberine must be taken with advice of ayurveda consultant. These natural extracts are not a replacement your diabetes medications. But they they contribute to better recovery and prevention as they have curative in nature.

Part-C

Exercise and Diabetes

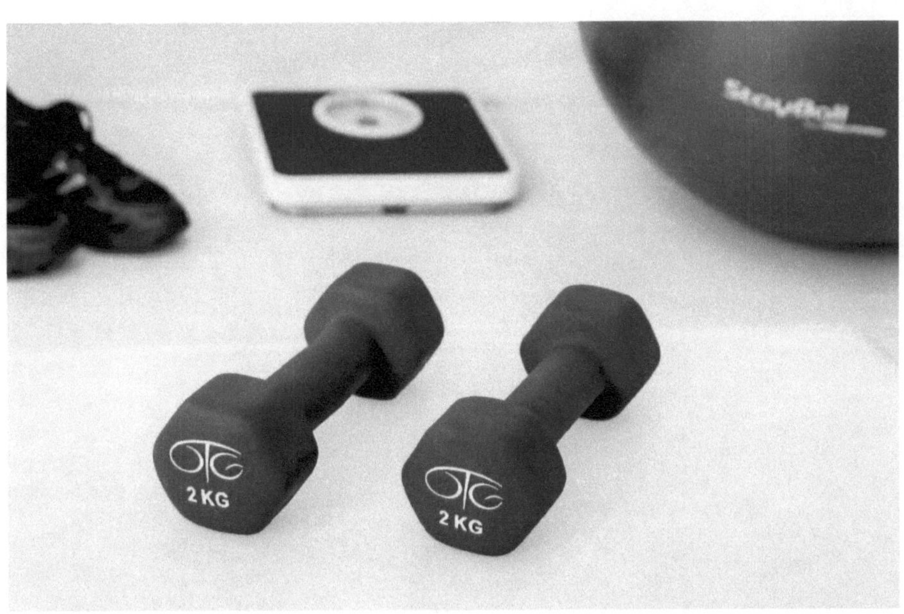

Chapter 1

Why Exercise Is Important for Diabetes

This chapter will dwell on the below two questions on exercises for diabetes.

WHY EXERCISE IS IMPORTANT FOR DIABETICS?

WHICH ARE BEST RECOMMEND EXERCISES FOR DIABETICS?

Most people know exercise is good but hardly few people do it consistently. Unlike smoking and alcohol People are not addicted to exercise because gratification is delayed in the latter and faster in former.

> "The doctor of the future will give no medicine, but will involve the patient in the proper use of food, fresh air and exercise."
>
> **– Thomas Edison**

In fact this was the case in in Ancient India, Vaidyas involved patients in the proper use of food, 5 elements and the nature. And also knowledge of the body and mind held by a common man in those days were far more superior than what we today know about our own body.

WHY EXERCISE IS MUST FOR DIABETICS?

Muscles can use glucose without insulin when exercising. That means Exercise makes the muscle to utilise glucose without the help of insulin. This is the biggest benefit of exercise for diabetics.

BENEFITS OF EXERCISE FOR DIABETICS:

1. Lowers blood sugar level.

2. Increases insulin sensitivity so that insulin acts better to control sugars.

3. It lowers blood pressure.

4. Lowers basal and postprandial insulin concentration.

5. Lowers Glycosylated hemoglobin (Hba1c).

6. Improves cholesterol levels.

7. Improves functioning of heart (cardiovascular system).

8. Increases strength and flexibility of joints.

9. Burns fat.

10. Reduces psychological stress by the action of endorphins.

11. Increases self esteem.

TIPS TO EXERCISE SAFELY:

1. Ideally, it is better to check blood sugars before exercise. If the fasting blood sugar is less than 85 mg per dl or random sugar more than 300 per dl, avoid exercise.

2. In the early morning, it is better to have 100 gm of fruit or low sugar protein shake before exercise.

3. Always exercise moderately.

4. Drink sips of water to avoid dehydration.

BEST EXERCISES FOR DIABETICS:

1. Brisk walking

2. Weight training

3. yoga

4. Swimming

5. stationary cycling

6. Tai-chi

Chapter 2

Is Only Walking Enough for Diabetics?

Walking is the simplest and easiest exercise. Most people follow walking as a form of Exercise. Many people walk as per their convenience and availability of time. Most Diabetic people walk regularly. However most of them are not aware of how much walking is required for effective blood sugar control.

HOW MUCH WALKING IS REQUIRED FOR DIABETICS?

IS IT 4400 STEPS (3.3 km), 6000 STEPS (4.6km) OR 10000 STEPS (7.6km)/DAY?.

Some studies suggest 4400 steps (3.3km) is good enough for optimum sugar control and it has shown to reduce Hba1c by 0.4%. Many type 2 diabetes people are overweight. To have a benefit of weight loss along with blood sugar control,10K steps or 7.6km walking per day is a must.

WHY 10k STEPS? WHY NOT 9k or 11K STEPS?

10000 steps is a magic number. Research has shown 10k is more beneficial than 9k and 11k steps walking doesn't give any additional benefits.

10k steps walking help in

a. Weight loss

b. Reducing Insulin resistance (it is the primary cause of type 2 diabetes and obesity)

c. It gives all other benefits of exercise.

HOW TO COUNT STEPS?

Walking 7.6 km or 10000 steps daily or atleast 5 days a week is not a easy job. It needs patience and perseverance. Easiest way to monitor steps is PEDOMETERS. It is now available on smartphones, fitness wrist bands and smart watches.

HOW TO PREPARE FOR A WALK?

Always use good quality walking shoes which supports the arch of the feet and which is flexible. Get socks made of fabrics like coolmax that wick away sweat and prevent blisters. Wear loose comfortable dress. Walk with head up and in a comfortable straight posture. During the first 10 minutes of walk, start with slow pace to warm up.

Attaining, 10k steps in walk on the very first day may not be possible for all. Start with 3k steps a day then improve it 5 to 6 k over next two weeks and finally 10k steps. Always try to walk in slow and fast pace alternately. Walking in company of friends will be motivating and entertaining. For a regular and long term practice, find a 'walk buddy.'

WHAT IF YOU CAN'T WALK DUE TO ARTHRITIS PROBLEM?

This is a common reason sighted by many people who are suffering from joint problems due to diabetes. Studies say nearly 50% people avoid walking because of arthritis issues. Please remember, Mild to moderate arthritis is not a reason to stop Walking. On the contrary Walking stabilizes muscles and bones. People with moderate arthritis must walk at least 20 to 25 min with a break in between. People with severe arthritis may opt for other exercises like stationary cycling, yoga, swimming or resistance training.

Only Walking is not enough. 2 days Weight training per week is required for better Diabetes control and to avoid age related muscle loss after the age of 40. We will look at aspects of weight training for diabetics in our next chapter.

Chapter 3

Weight Training/Resistance Training for Diabetics

Most of type 2 diabetes patients in india, especially those above 45 to 50 years of age adopt only WALKING as a mode of exercise. Few of them practice other aerobic exercise like cycling, swimming etc. Very few diabetic people in india after 50 hit the gym for weight training. I hardly see woman above 40s opting for weight training. Many women in india feel resistance training is not for them. It is important for both men and women to maintain lean toned muscles.

Aerobic training (walking, cycling, swimming etc) involves continuous activity of multiple large muscle groups, whereas strength training involves isolated, brief but intense activity of single muscle groups. After the age of 35, there is 3% muscle loss every year. To maintain muscle mass after 35 years, resistance training is very essential.

Benefits of Resistance training for diabetics:

1. Resistance training actually improves insulin sensitivity better than aerobic exercises.

2. Toned muscles also use glucose more effectively, and that helps regulate blood sugar even when you're at rest.

3. Strength training also helps build stronger bones, thus helps in preventing osteoporosis.

4. As you age, strength training (also called resistance training), gives more stamina to do everyday activities such as walking, lifting things, and climbing stairs etc.

5. Strength training also helps in decreasing the amount of insulin utilised by your body to store energy in fat cells, thus considerably reducing your fat-to-muscle ratio.

6. Strength training leads to an increase in muscle mass. This raises your Basal Metabolic Rate and causes the body to burn more calories naturally.

7. More muscles – more mitochondria – much younger you look and rate of ageing decreases.

Weekly twice strength training is very much essential for diabetics.

Combining 3 days of aerobic exercises with 2 days of weight training per week is more beneficial in controlling blood sugars and achieving HBa1c targets.

BASIC strength training Exercises

- Planks, squats and lunges.

- Standing biceps curl.

- Triceps extension.

- shoulder presses.

- chest press.

- classic crunches.

- Spend enough time on warming up and mobilizing the target joint and muscles involved in the workouts for the day.

- Optimise workout intensity with help of a fitness trainer. A person trainer is always better to have.

- Use a mix of weights machines and resistance bands for the training.

NOTE: Having 100 g fruit is a good option before strength training exercises. Or, having fruit based smoothie without sugar is also ideal before workout.

If your diabetes is uncontrolled or have fluctuating sugar levels, blood sugar monitoring must be done before and after exercise so that accordingly you can eat what is required to be eaten pre and post workout

Caution: Strength training is not advisable for people with Diabetes retinopathy where vision may be impaired and for those with severe comorbidity like chronic kidney diseases, stroke etc.

Chapter 4

Swimming for Diabetes

Swimming is perfect exercise for whole body. It increases flexibility, muscle strength and endurance. It is an exercise which doesn't make you sweat. It is an exercise which can be done by people suffering from arthritis. Swimming is good exercise for kids as well as old age persons.

Four reasons why diabetics must swim:

1. It burns more calories than running:

   One hour of vigorous lap swimming can burn as much as 700 calories.

   The same amount of time running at 5 mph burns only 600 calories.

2. Swimming helps to sleep better:

   Many old age people are suffering from insomnia.

   Swimming have the power to help you sleep better at night.

3. Swimming is a good exercise for lungs and heart:

   It is one of the exercises recommended for exercise-induced asthma where in other exercises can aggregate asthma symptoms.

   It is also good for cardiovascular health.

4. Swimming is good for depression and stress:

   Swimming is relaxing and elevates mood.

   It is good to swim at least twice a week in a clean water.

Part-D

Ancient Secrets to Prevent and Reverse Diabetes

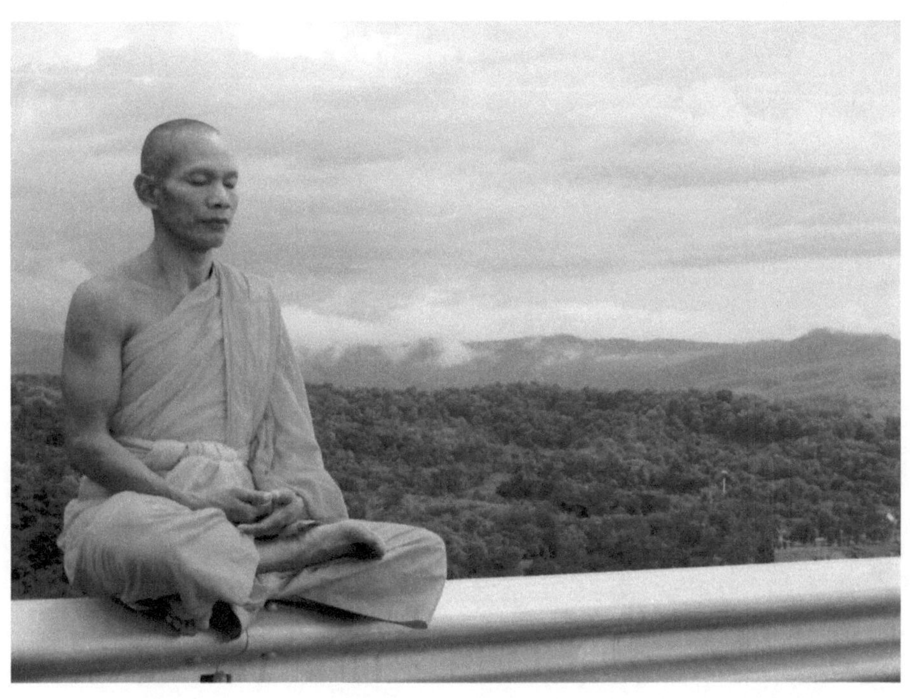

Chapter 1

How Yoga Helps Diabetes!

Yoga is one of the best recommended exercises for diabetes. In fact it is much more than an exercise, if done with awareness and learnt from a proper Acharya, yoga will help you maximize every aspect of your life. Yoga can make you get in touch with the healer within you. Yoga is a series of mental, physical and breathing discipline that originated in ancient India and deals with every aspect of body, mind and soul.

Yoga offers a multifaceted solution for the treatment of Diabetes. Modern studies have proved and recognized that Diabetes responds very well to Yogic management.

Here are 5 WAYS YOGA HELPS IN DIABETES Management and Reversal

Diabetes is a condition which occurs either due to lack of insulin production by the pancreas or lack of cell response to insulin. Blood sugars in diabetes can also be deranged by daily stress levels and chronic stress.

1. Yoga asanas makes abdominal contractions and release, which stimulates the pancreas, increasing blood and oxygen supply. The pancreatic cells, buffeted by fresh blood flow, undergo a rejuvenation that increases the ability to produce insulin.

2. Some yoga postures, pranayama and meditation has shown to encourage proper functioning of the endocrine glands.

3. Yoga also increases glucose uptake by muscular cells, which in turn, decreases insulin resistance which helps to lower blood sugar levels.

4. Yoga can relieve you from daily stress factors which usually increase blood sugar levels, hence Yoga helps in reducing blood sugars due to chronic stress.

5. Regular yoga practice with awareness can help in focussing and create the right mental attitude necessary for diabetes management and reversal.

Yogic management of diabetes includes the practice of:

1. Satwika-aahaara (Yogic diet).

2. Asanas (postures).

3. Kriyas (Cleansing techniques).

4. Pranayamas (breathing practices) and Bandhas/neuromuscular locks.

5. Meditation.

Opting for any one of them exclusively or in combination, helps in diabetes management and reversal provided you are making the practice an integral part of your life with great reverence and gratitude.

*Thanks for the inputs from Vijayalakshmi Pai.

Chapter 2

Best Yogasanas for Diabetes

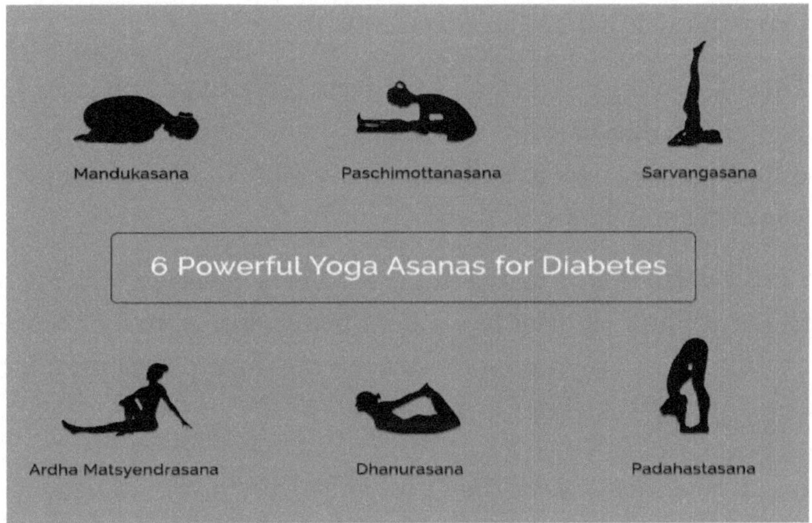

This "6 posture program" is a well-balanced Asana module that's target specific and addresses all major factors that instigate Diabetes – stress, dysfunctional Pancreas, insulin resistance etc.

1. Padahastasana:

   It's a deep forward bending pose practiced in standing position.

   Creates squeezing effect on the pancreas which results in rich blood flow to it.

   Rich blood flow rectifies insulin secretory functioning of the pancreas

   NOTE: Contraindicated for pregnancy.

2. Ardha Matsyendrasana:

   This is a potential twisting pose in seated position; one of the most efficient and clinically proven Asanas for diabetes. This asana specifically targets and stimulates pancreas aiding its rejuvenation. Stimulates blood circulation to pancreas and restores its capacity to produce insulin.

   NOTE: Contraindicated for pregnancy.

3. Paschimottanasana:

   This is a classical Asana with deep forward bending in seated position. Achieves deep massaging of the abdominal organs and stimulates the pancreas. The compression it causes on pancreas results in more blood flow to it.

   Classical reference, Hatha-Yoga-Pradipika mentions that it treats all the abdominal disorders, aiding better digestion. It is helpful in treating classical symptoms of diabetes, such as polyphagia.

4. Dhanurasana:

   It's an intense back bending pose practiced in face-down position. Massages and tones the abdominal organs directly. Strengthens back muscles and enhances toning of abdominal viscera (muscles & vital organs including pancreas)

   NOTE: Contraindications – Pregnancy and severe lower back pain

5. Mandukasana:

   A simple forward bending posture with Brahma-mudra practiced in Vajrasana position; one among the most essential postures in treating diabetes. Improves blood supply to the pancreas by massaging and toning the abdominal area. It activates pancreas and improves the quantity of insulin production.

   NOTE: not recommended for pregnant women

6. Sarvangasana:

   Best inversion posture to treat Diabetes! It revitalizes and regulates the functioning of all the endocrine glands including pancreas. It increases metabolic activity in the body ensuring optimal utilization of insulin; Treats the symptom of insulin resistance and improves blood circulation all over the body.

   NOTE: Contraindications – Pregnancy and complications of diabetes such as heart ailments etc.

The other 3 powerful Yoga practices for diabetes are:

- Kapalabhati

- Agnisara Kriya

- Surya namaskar

1. KAPALABHATI:

Its a power breath practice where exhalation happens actively & inhalation passively. Active contraction of abdominal muscles stimulates & tones the pancreas and restores secretory functions. Purifies toxics from the body and reduces internal inflammation. It balances both Kapha & Pitta doshas, thereby ensuring optimal functioning of Insulin in the whole body. Kapalabhati is to be done in the morning empty stomach.

Kapalabhati is very powerful in purifying our internal system, improves gut health, increases alertness and ability become aware of what is happening with is and around,

2. AGNISARA KRIYA:

It involves continuous flapping of abdominal muscles. Tones and massages the abdomen muscles ensuring rich blood flow to the pancreas. It stimulates and activates the pancreatic gland & improves insulin secretory function.

3. SURYANAMASKAR: (12 poses)

It involves the movement of the whole body. It improves the functioning of pancreas and also improves insulin sensitivity. Suryanamaskara is to be done consistently, correctly with a sense of gratitude. Lethargy and laziness will be out of our systems. Ability to think clearly enhances. Keeps nerve systems healthy, muscles and tendons healthy and strong. It absorbs cosmic energy into our cells and activates healing. It can keep you energetic always and reduces dependence on food. There are yogis in India, who do 108 to 512

Suryanamaskaras everyday and just live on water and on some days just a simple meal once.

Ideally if Suryanamaskara is done 24 times at a stretch it is even better than doing a high intensity strength and conditioning exercise or high intensity cardio. Please Note Suryanamaskara must end by the time Sun rises or within 15 minutes of the sunrise.

Sun is the Lifeforce of our Solar System and Surya Namaskara is a way to channelize the cosmic energy and regulates the various prana elements in the body.

***NOTE*:** Readers are requested to practice these techniques under expert guidance. It is also essential to be personally instructed as to how and when to perform them according to individual needs.

Yoga when practiced well, rejuvenate the organs cells and regulates stress hormones which is a important for good blood sugar control. From a yogic perspective it regulates various energy centers and systems in our body.

It is perfect Mind – Body phenomenon and beyond.

Chapter 3

Tai-Chi for Diabetics

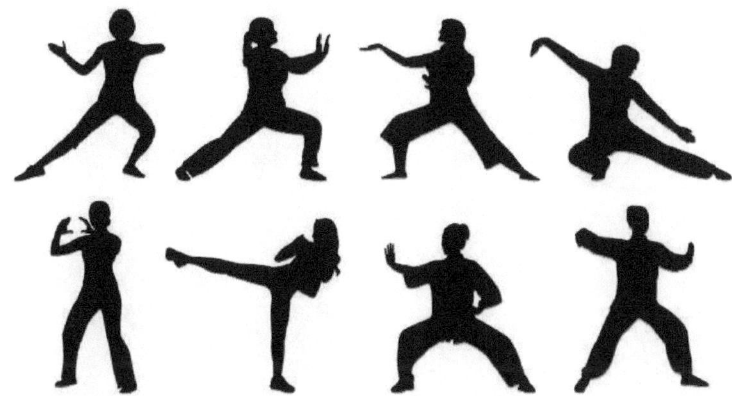

Tai chi is an ancient Chinese tradition that, today, is practiced as a form of exercise. It involves a series of movements performed in a slow, focused manner and accompanied by deep breathing.

Since ancient times Chinese people have been practicing to tai chi for longevity and its other benefits.

Tai chi is low impact and puts minimal stress on muscles and joints, making it generally safe for all ages.

Benefits of Tai-chi:

❖ Decreased stress, and anxiety.

❖ Improved mood.

❖ Improved aerobic capacity.

❖ Increased energy and stamina.

❖ Improves flexibility, and balance.

❖ Improved muscle strength.

Thus, Tai-chi is also one of the best recommended exercise for diabetics.

Chapter 4

10 Ways Meditation Helps in Diabetes Control

Medical science has made tremendous progress in last 30 years in terms of treating infections, trauma management, advances in surgeries like, keyhole surgeries, robotic surgeries etc but have failed to control the rise of Diabetes.

Though there are many discoveries on new diabetes medicines and newer types of insulin, LIFESTYLE CHANGES are the key in the management of diabetes. Somehow the significant role of lifestyle is ignored by the most.

Diabetes management needs BALANCE:

- Balance in Diet and eating.

- Balance in Exercise and activity.

- Balance in stress and sleep.

"Meditation is the key tool in bringing about a balance in lifestyle, energies within and the proportion of Satva, Rajas and Tamas – the various states of activity in a person."

By accepting Diabetes and being fully aware of how life and the management of diabetes transact, one can learn to manage diabetes effectively and if consistent reversal is possible too.

HOW MEDITATION HELPS IN BLOOD SUGAR CONTROL?

Meditation helps in lowering blood sugar by

1. Reducing chronic inflammation in the body.

2. Increasing insulin production (study in Massachusetts general hospital).

3. Increasing mitochondrial metabolism (power centres of cells).

4. Altering genetic expression i.e Epigenetics (observed in long term meditators). Good genes which regulates endocrine system gets switched on, this keeps the endocrine system which regulate an array hormones, healthy.

5. By reducing stress hormones. Meditation reduces stress hormones and prevents stress induced increase of blood sugars.

6. Meditation decreases CRAVINGS:

   Many Diabetics have cravings for sugar and other unhealthy food choices. This craving will disappear with continuous practice of meditation

7. Meditation relieves CHRONIC PAIN:

   Many Diabetics are suffering from nerve pains in legs (peripheral neuropathy). Meditation is helpful in reducing chronic pains and unpleasant sensations.

8. Cures INSOMNIA:

   Old Diabetics have problem in sleeping. Disturbed sleep increases stress hormones, which increases blood sugar levels. Meditation helps in improving quality of sleep.

9. Meditation is known to help in reducing Cardiovascular vascular complications: Heart attacks and increase in Blood pressure are known complications of Diabetes. Meditation helps in reducing BP and also decreases Heart attack risks.

10. Meditation is very much required to effectively manage Gestational diabetes. (Diabetes in pregnancy) Along with controlling sugars, it helps in reducing stress and anxiety related to pregnancy.

Consistently practice meditation technique you know for at least 1 hr in a day.

Some of the meditation techniques which are of great help in diabetes are

1. Mindfulness Meditation.

2. Transcendental meditation.

3. Solar plexus chakra meditation.

Chapter 5

Fasting to Cure Diabetes

Do You Know "Planned Fasting Is Effective In Prevention And Reversal Of Diabetes."

Don't get scared of fasting.

Fasting is not starvation.

Fasting is only time restricted eating.

Above all fasting is safely time tested from thousands of years in all religions of the world.

Many case studies and research has shown that fasting is effective in reducing insulin resistance and thereby prevention and reversal of type 2 diabetes.

As far back as 1916, Dr. Joslin one of the Famous diabetes specialist of this century reported the benefits of fasting for Diabetes. Fasting is the most efficient and consistent strategy to decrease insulin levels and break Insulin resistance. This is now widely accepted as true through various research and findings from experiments and also results through clinical practices.

This is how fasting helps in Diabetes

When we eat food, blood sugar rises and so insulin rises to control blood sugars. When fasting, there is no blood sugar rise and hence no insulin rise. During fasting, we first burn glycogen stored in the liver. When that is consumed by the body, we use body fat.

Glucose and fat are main sources of energy for the body. If glucose is not available, then the body will adjust and generate energy by burning fat, without any detrimental health effects, as it is body's natural mechanism. Intermittent Fasting in addition to lowering insulin levels has also been shown to improve insulin sensitivity significantly. (by breaking insulin resistance)

Fasting is better than consuming 5 to 6 six small portion meals with calorie restriction. Calorie restricted diet over a long time slows down body metabolism and leads to loss of lean muscle mass.

Fasting boosts basal metabolism and preserves lean muscle mass.

Which is better for reversal of diabetes? – >Low carbohydrate-healthy fat diet or fasting?

Both FASTING and low-carbohydrate, healthy-fat (LCHF) diets effectively can cause weight loss and reverse type 2 diabetes. Fasting lowers insulin faster and most efficiently. Very low–carbohydrate diet gives 70% percent of the benefits of the fasting without actual fasting. Combining intermittent fasting with low carbohydrates diet is always the best option.

Chapter 6

How to Do Fasting When Taking Diabetes Medications?

When you start fasting with change of diet, it requires adjustment of diabetes medications by your physician or diabetologist. If dose adjustments are not done as per the diabetic status of the person chances of hypoglycaemia (low sugar) can be common. Some diabetes drugs, like insulin and sulfonylureas are known to cause hypoglycemia. It is better to avoid them when on fasting or low carbohydrates diet.

Metformin, DPP-4 inhibitors, and SGL T2 inhibitors have a lower risk of hypoglycemia, so they can be preferred with dosage adjustments. When you are fasting with medications or insulin, monitoring of blood sugar is required 2 to 4 times daily. When fasting without medications, glucose monitoring is not required.

Other medications like Bp medicines can be taken during fasting. Some of gastric irritation medications like iron supplements, aspirin etc must be taken with advice of the physician.

Fasting regime is not same for all patients. Fasting duration vary from 16 hrs to 36 hrs. It must be done with supervision. People who are recently diagnosed with diabetes (or less than 5 years) respond well and reverse their diabetes within 4 to 6 months. People who were diabetic for more than 10 years take more time.

Patients with diabetes related complications like chronic kidney disease must follow fasting with proper supervision only.

Fasting is the natural way of preventing and reversing type 2 diabetes which is worth a try. In my clinical practice i have been able to reverse diabetes of many people through a combination of customised Intermittent Fasting, LCHF Diet or Keto Diet, Lifestyle Changes, Exercises & Yoga and Meditation.

Part-E

Gestational Diabetes

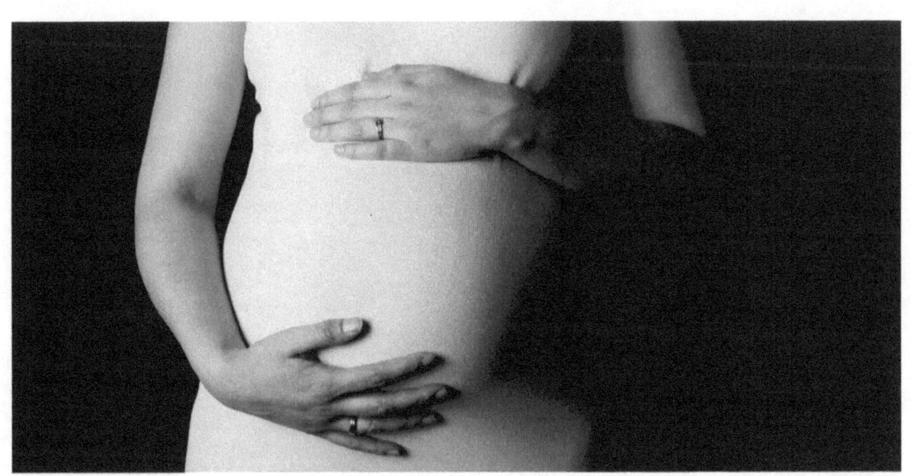

Chapter 1

Let Us Understand Gestational Diabetes

1 OUT OF 5 PREGNANT WOMEN IN INDIA HAVE DIABETES.

Gestational Diabetes develop during pregnancy cause high blood sugar levels and in extreme cases harm the baby. An estimated 5 million women develop GDM every year. Although GDM is a temporary phenomenon for the pregnant woman, more than 50% of women with GDM develop Type 2 Diabetes within 5–10 years of delivery. Also the chances of their children being diabetic increases, later in their adulthood.

Not all women develop GDM. Why it affects only few women is not completely known.

During pregnancy, the placenta brings about many hormonal changes, thereby impacting the action of insulin, raising your blood sugar levels.

WHAT ARE THE RISK FACTORS OF GDM?

1. Pregnant women above the age of 35 yrs.

2. Family history of GDM.

3. Presence of Prediabetes.

4. Overweight or Obese women.

When to screen for GDM?

IT IS RECOMMENDED TO SCREEN FOR DIABETES FROM 24 TO 28 WEEKS OF PREGNANCY.

Once diagnosed with GDM, its advisable to follow the below religiously–

1. MONITOR BLOOD SUGAR LEVELS REGULARLY. Many apparatuses are available in the market to test for blood sugar at home. Target range of blood sugar is lower for pregnancy diabetes.

2. SWITCH TO LOW CARBOHYDRATES-HEALTHY FAT DIET.

Limit your intake of highly refined carbs like bread, wheat, white rice and sweets.

It is good to have lot of vegetables with healthy natural fats with limited quantity of fruits.

There is a cultural tendency to eat more fruits during pregnancy.

Too much of fruits will rise blood sugar levels

3. REGULAR PHYSICAL ACTIVITIES/EXERCISES:

Exercise lowers the levels of blood sugar by stimulating the body to move glucose into cells. As an added bonus, regular exercises also help alleviate other pregnancy and delivery related complications like back pain, muscle cramps and swelling.

4. TREATMENT:

Most often insulin is offered as treatment for GDM. In few cases oral drugs like metformin is recommended. Remember GDM can be prevented if proper weight and diet is maintained before pregnancy.

Chapter 2

10 Known Complications of Poorly Controlled Gestational Diabetes Mellitus?

Complications of untreated and uncontrolled blood sugars occur to both mother and Babies. 10 complications of Gestational DIABETES everyone must know are as below:

1. LARGE BABIES

   High glucose can cross the placenta, which makes baby's pancreas to make extra insulin. This extra insulin can cause baby to grow too large, a condition called MACROSOMIA.

2. Babies May develop LOW SUGARS immediately after birth.

3. PREGNANT DIABETIC MOTHERS (GDM) May develop High blood pressure condition called PREECLAMPSIA.

4. Gestational diabetes, high blood sugar condition during pregnancy, may cause early-stage KIDNEY damage that can later lead to chronic kidney diseases among women.

5. GESTATIONAL DIABETIC MOTHERS are at high risk of developing Diabetes in next pregnancy and in later life.

6. UNCONTROLLED AND UNTREATED high blood sugars in pregnancy may lead to death of the baby rarely.

7. Babies born to diabetic mothers have high risk of developing obesity and type 2 diabetes later in life.

8. Researchers found that women with a history of gestational diabetes had a 40% percent greater risk of developing cardiovascular diseases like Heart attacks and stroke.

9. Gestational Diabetic Mothers have higher chance of going for Caesarean sections because of large babies

10. Gestational Diabetic Mothers have risk of early-preterm births.

All pregnant women and family must be aware of the potential complications of Gestational DIABETES. It is advisable for pregnant diabetic women to control their blood sugars with regular follow up with Diabetologist and physician.

Part-F

Myths and Uncommon Facts on Diabetes

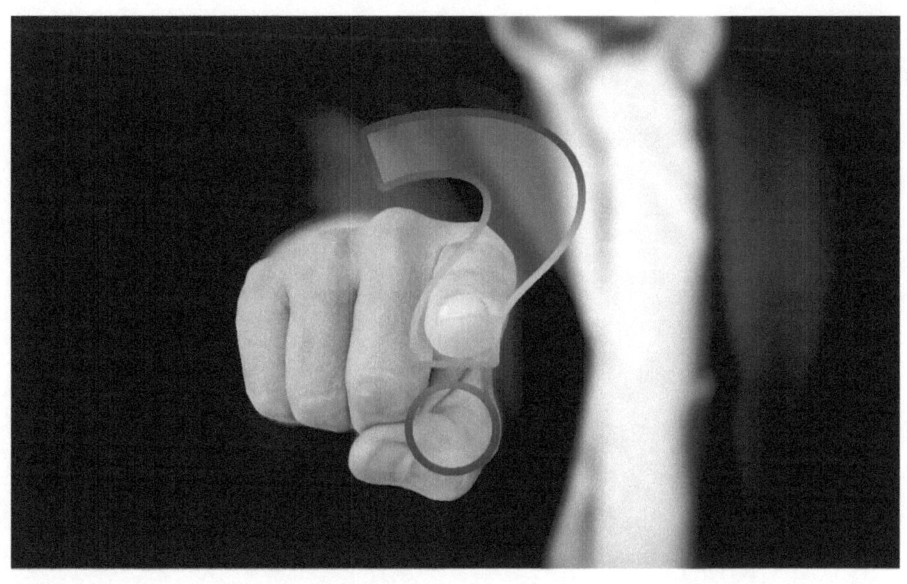

Chapter 1

Stress Can Spike Sugars

Many chronic health problems of this century are due to stress and sugar. Stress increases the risk of developing diabetes and worsens the existing diabetes condition. Chronic stress impacts blood sugar levels directly. Along with good diet and exercise, stress management is equally important in Diabetes control and reversal.

As seen in my clinical practice, sugars go high due to stress alone despite people following proper diet and exercise. It is so influencing that chronic stress alters blood glucose levels in 4 ways

1. Stress hormone like cortisol increases blood sugar levels.

2. People in stress fail to take care of their diet and lifestyle and often binge eat leading to high blood sugars.

3. Stress can actually cause many people to accumulate more belly fat. More the chronic stress, more is the amount of cortisol is in your body and more the abdominal fat. Increase in abdominal fat increase the risk of developing diabetes as well as worsen existing diabetic conditions in the body.

4. Stress contributes to insulin resistance. Thus, managing stress is a essential part of diabetes control and reversal. Sometimes it is difficult to manage stress living in a 24 by 7 internet addicted and sleepless society.

Chapter 2

9 Common Diabetes Myths

1. **Rice Is Bad for Diabetes and wheat chapatis are safe – Not True.**

   Though white rice is bad for diabetes, red, black or brown rices are better for diabetics in small quantities. Wheat is also a refined carbohydrate. It is better to avoid all refined carbohydrates like white rice, wheat, maida, rawa and sugars.

2. **Fasting Is Not Good For Diabetes – Not True.**

   Intermittent Fasting on the advice and supervision of the doctor helps in reducing insulin resistance. Medications do need to be adjusted depending on the time of fasting

Fasting Benefits in diabetes are

   a. Improved insulin sensitivity.

   b. Lowered triglycerides.

   c. Weight loss.

   d. Normalises prediabetes.

   e. In some cases, can help in the reversal of diabetes.

Intermittent fasting is the best dietary intervention for prediabetes or borderline diabetes.

3. **Diabetes Is A Chronic Progressive Disease – Not True.**

   Type 2 Diabetes although widely believed to be a chronic progressive disease, is reversible in many cases. Recent cases studies and examples proved many Type 2 diabetes are effectively reversible with low carbohydrates diet and fasting.

4. **Insulin Is Needed Only In Later Stage And Severe Diabetes – Not True.**

   In type 2 diabetes, insulin treatment cause weight gain and further worsens the diabetic condition. Insulin can be used in the treatment for diabetics even in early stages if the sugars are very high or are with any comorbid complications. A recent study suggested that insulin is a good choice if a person's HbA1c levels remain above 8% while only on oral tablets, i.e., even within 3–4 months of diagnosis.

5. **Diabetes Cannott Be Reversed – Not True.**

Type 1 diabetes is not reversible.

Many cases of Type 2 Diabetes can be reversed by conforming to low carbohydrate diet, fasting and lifestyle.

6. **Artificial sweeteners are safe to use in diabetes.**

Artificial sweeteners may not increase the blood sugars levels. But, excessive use of sweeteners are not good for health.

7. **Low fat diet is helpful in diabetes – Not true.**

LCHF Diet is a required for diabetes management and reversal. As discussed in the earlier chapters fat is the least stimulant of insulin secretion and fat doesn't raise blood sugars like carbohydrates.

8. **Fruits are healthy, so one can eat fruits as many: Not true.**

Fruits have natural sugars. They tend to rise blood sugars. Fruits must be consumed in moderation in diabetes.

9. **If you are not experiencing any signs of diabetes, you are fine and need not worry: Not true.**

Many a times diabetes with moderate to high sugars doesn't show immediate symptoms. Poorly controlled diabetes keeps damaging the body from inside. It is always better to monitor symptoms irrespectively.

Usual and Unusual Signs and Symptoms of Type 2 Diabetes Mellitus Unique to Men and Women

As seen in my clinical practice, few people who are diagnosed to have type 2 diabetes are symptomless without any specific complaints. The classical signs and symptoms of diabetes need not be there in all patients.

Some people have classical common symptoms of diabetes which is easy to diagnose whereas, some people have unusual rare symptoms which give only clue or suspicion of diabetes.

Since Diabetes is rapidly rising since last decade, it is essential for all to know the signs and symptoms of diabetes which helps in early detection and treatment.

The COMMON signs and symptoms of diabetes are:

1. Increased thirst

2. Frequent urination

3. Increased hunger

4. Tiredness

5. Unexpected weight loss

6. Blurring of vision

The UNUSUAL or LESS COMMON signs and symptoms of Diabetes are:

1. Frequent infections:

   Diabetes leads to low immune status. Low immune status leads to frequent infections. Since Yeasts (fungus) and Bacteria multiply in high numbers in presence of sugars, frequent infections are common in diabetes.

2. Slow healing wounds:

   High blood sugar decreases the amount of oxygen delivered to wounds through the bloodstream which slows down the healing process.

3. Darkening of skin:

    Dark, velvety patches in the folds of skin, usually on the back of neck, knuckles, and elbows are often early warning signs of high blood sugar. High insulin levels increase melanin levels and make skin look dark.

4. Improvements in vision:

    High blood sugar in Diabetes causes the shift of fluid levels including the lenses of eyes, leading to a change of refractive power and change in power of glasses indicating a better vision.

    This sometimes lead to improvement in vision and negates the need for glasses. When blood sugars are controlled on treatment, again refractive errors of the eye are normalised to previous levels and one would need glasses again.

5. Tingling and numbness in limbs:

    High blood sugars cause nerve damage leading to tingling and numbness sensations in limbs.

6. Itching of skin:

    Diabetes impairs blood circulation and can lead to dryness and itching.

7. Decreased hearing:

    Hearing loss could be an early sign of diabetes. Diabetes damage the blood vessels and nerves of the inner ear leading to decreased hearing.

8. Increase in snoring:

    One study confirmed 23% of sleep apnea which is characterized by loud snoring and daytime sleepiness will develop diabetes in the next 5 years.

People with disordered breathing, tend to release stress hormones during sleep which can lead to an increase in blood sugars.

9. Sexual issues:

High blood sugar can cause damage to blood vessels and nerves that are needed for normal sexual response leading to sexual dysfunction in both men and women.

UNIQUE SIGNS AND SYMPTOMS OF DIABETES IN MEN:

Apart from above common signs and symptoms, men can have

1. Erectile dysfunction – It is the inability of a man to achieve or maintain an erection. According to a recent meta-analysis of 140 studies, 50% of men with Type 2 Diabetes are suffering from erectile dysfunction.

2. Retrograde ejaculation:

Semen instead of ejecting outside is being released back into the urinary bladder. Thus very less semen gets released during sexual ejaculation.

3. Urological issues like hyperactive bladder, inability to control urine and urine infections. Urological issues can happen due to diabetic nerve damage.

SIGNS AND SYMPTOMS UNIQUE TO WOMEN ARE:

1. Vaginal itching and fungal infections.

2. Lower sexual drive and some cases lead to painful sex.

3. Frequent urine infections.

The cause of the above 3 symptoms of diabetes in women has been explained above.

4. Polycystic ovarian syndrome (PCOS).

Women with PCOS are at greater risk of diabetes. Symptoms of PCOS are irregular cycles, weight gain, and acne along with fertility problems. PCOS leads to insulin resistance which in turn causes diabetes.

All diabetic people and their family members must have knowledge of the signs and symptoms of diabetes which help in early detection of high blood sugar and its complications.

Chapter 4

13 Must Know Interesting Facts about Diabetes

1. Since there is increase in urine frequency while DIABETIC, it was considered a kidney disease till 18th century.

2. Diabetes is a disease of the whole body. It is not just a blood sugar disease.

3. Excess glucose attracts fungal infections.

   Thus fungal infections are common in uncontrolled diabetes.

4. Diabetics lose weight in spite of heightened hunger. Since insulin is not acting due to insulin resistance, brain starts using fat and muscle leading to weight loss.

5. BITTER GOURD is good for diabetics as it's seeds contain insulin.

6. CINNAMON is good for diabetics as it activates enzymes that help in insulin absorption

7. Type 2 DIABETES is a completely reversible condition. It is not a permanent, chronic progressive disease.

8. DAWN phenomenon – It means high fasting sugars and normal sugars after breakfast. Growth hormone secretion in early morning leads to high Fasting blood sugars which gets normal after breakfast.

9. SOMAGYI EFFECT:

   Sometimes Insulin or Diabetes medication acts too strongly in the night between 2am to 3 am which leads to a low sugar then sugar level rise due to compensatory mechanisms.

10. Indian physicians sushrutha and charaka mentioned about the difference between type 1 and type 2 diabetes in 400 to 500 CE.

11. Women with polycystic ovaries (PCOD) are at greater risk of developing diabetes.

12. New research is linking diabetes to air pollution and other pollutants which causes inflammation that gradually triggers Diabetes.

13. PROBIOTICS HELPS DIABETES CONTROL:

Probiotics are a kind of bacteria found in our gut that can help with digestion. Consumption of Probiotic rich foods or probiotic supplements are highly beneficial in reducing insulin resistance is Type 2 diabetes.

Chapter 5

How to Prevent Diabetes If There Is a Strong Family History or Genetic Risk of Type 2 Diabetes?

There are hereditary as well as genetic factors which influence the occurrence of type 2 Diabetes.

If both parents are diabetic, there is 50% more risk of developing Diabetes.

If one parent is diabetic, there is 25% risk of developing diabetes.

With good lifestyle and diet, genetic expressions can be altered to a great extent.

Factors which affect the gene expression include diet, quality of sleep, exercise, yoga, breathing techniques, emotions, and meditation.

All of these things will influence the gene expression.

"This new science is called the epi-genetics," says Deepak Chopra.

By following healthy lifestyle and diet explained in this chapter, even genetic and hereditary risk of type 2 diabetes can be prevented to great extent.

Sometimes type 2 diabetes run in families not because of genes but because of lifestyle,

This tendency is due to children learning bad eating habits from their parents—eating a poor diet, not exercising—and leading a poor lifestyle.

Gene can determine our potential but they can't determine our destiny. Whatever is the associated risk, focus on healthy lifestyle.

Conclusion

Diabetes and obesity are like modern day slow plague. Both Diabetes and obesity incidences have almost quadrupled since 1980. Obesity is the precursor to the development of diabetes, though many thin individuals also develop diabetes.

Poorly regulated food industry, less emphasis on food and diet by medical systems and governments too are responsible for this menace. Unfortunately there is no reversal option for type 1 diabetes, which primarily affects children and there is a deficiency of insulin in the body.

In type 2 diabetes is caused in 90% cases by insulin resistance and hyperinsulinemia.

High carbohydrates diet, sugars, processed foods, stress are the main reasons behind insulin resistance. Genetics and hereditary factors play a minor role in causation of type 2 diabetes.

When we focus on factors which causes hyperinsulinemia and insulin resistance, type 2 diabetes can be reversed.

Traditionally people used to eat lot of healthy fats, real unrefined carbohydrates and proteins since ages.

In last 50 years food technology advances and food guidelines recommended low fat diets which created real problems.

Low fat guidelines created a "fat phobia "in people's mind.

People stopped eating fats.

Natural fats are building blocks of body and least stimulants of insulin.

By avoiding fats, people started consuming more refined carbohydrates like sugars, Maida, white rice, wheat, rawa, pasta, breads etc.

Carbohydrates rich diet increases hyperinsulinemia and insulin resistance which is the primary cause of type 2 diabetes.

Along with unhealthy refined carbohydrates rich diet, people were more exposed to processed foods pressures (stress) of modern life and pollution.

People neglected ancient health principles like 1) not eating late in the night 2) Eating real raw foods 3) living stress free with meditation 4) mind body exercises like yoga and pranayama.

All these factors are responsible for explosion of diabetes epidemic.

If we don't ring an alert now, we will end up in creating generations of people with diabetes.

WHO predicted that by 2020, two third of health problems will be due to chronic lifestyle diseases. Diabetes and obesity are predominantly lifestyle diseases.

Reducing high blood sugars in diabetes is not the proper treatment.

Reducing high sugars with medications only symptomatic treatment.

It is like treating only fever in typhoid without killing the salmonella typhi bacteria which caused typhoid.

Proper treatment of diabetes must include managing high blood sugars along with trying to address the root cause which causes diabetes.

Lifestyle changes and dietary changes are helpful in addressing the root causes of diabetes not just medications or insulin. Yogic practices further help in healing and reversal.

Don't accept the fact that diabetes is progressive disease. it is reversible.

More awareness is needed for people. It is the combined responsibility of patients, doctors, healthcare system and governments to alert and address this fast growing epidemic.

More importantly it is the personal commitment to adhere to healthy lifestyle that makes a difference.

In the next section of this book I have included three Case studies of Diabetes Reversal from my clinical practice.

Case 1

Gaurav Sharma: 40 year old IT engineer by profession. He weighed 108 kg. He is hardworking and active. He was on two diabetes medications (Glimepiride and Metformin) and insulin. (Human Mixtard 15-0-15). In Spite of this his HBa1c was 10.5

His weight was constant since last 2 years. He was following calorie restricted diet which contained 70% carbohydrates.

I advised him to shift to low carbohydrate diet (less than 20% carbs) I reduced his insulin by 4 units every 15 days with glucose monitoring at home. I Changed his oral glimepiride – metformin combination to metformin-voglibose which is weight neutral.

Over a period of 2 months, I stopped his insulin and added SGLT 2 inhibitors. SGLT 2 inhibitors are diabetic drugs which helps in weight loss.

With low carbohydrates diet and change of medications, his weight reduced by 8 kgs in 3 months. His HBa1c reduced to 7.5 from 10.5 After 3 months, I put him on an intermittent fasting regimen.

After 3 months, his HBa1c recorded just 6.5. His weight got reduced by total 12 kgs. Now he is on only on metformin 500 twice a day.

Sometimes he does have challenges in following the low carbohydrate diet and fasting regimen due to his hectic work schedule. He follows it most of the times.

He is on the verge of diabetes reversal if he continues following the low carbohydrate diet, fasting and the exercise regimen.

Case 2

Nisha, 30 years,

A Dental doctor, diagnosed with Gestational Diabetes in her first pregnancy. She continues to have diabetes post pregnancy.

Her post pregnancy weight was 86 kg with BMI 29. For her diabetes, she consulted an Endocrinologist and started medications.

When she met me, she was on insulin three times – Insulin (Inj. Novorapid 18-18-18) and two diabetes medicines. (Sitagliptin 50 mg twice a day and metformin 1 gms twice a day). Her HBa1c was 8.5

She was following a calorie restricted diet. But her diet was predominantly rice based and carbohydrates rich. Protein intake was not adequate in her diet.

I counselled her on following a low carbohydrate diet and Exercise. I asked her to finish dinner before 7 pm.

After 2 weeks of starting low carbohydrate diet with adequate proteins and natural fats.

Her sugar levels started to dip. I gradually reduced her insulin doses. Over a period of two months her insulin consumption frequency was reduced to just 10 units once a day from thrice in a day. After another 3 months, she was taken off from her insulin injections completely.

Her weight reduced by 4 kgs in 3 months.

Her HBa1c reduced to 7.5

I changed her oral medications to SGLT 2 inhibitors and metformin.

She was instructed to follow 15 hrs intermittent fasting pattern.

Over the next 2 months, Her HbA1c dropped to 6.7% and weight reduced by another 2 kgs. Now she is on metformin 500 twice a day.

She is consistently following low carbohydrate diet, intermittent fasting-5 days a week and exercise. She too is on the verge of reversing her diabetes.

Case 3

Rajeev.

A Businessman

His weight is 70 kg, fit and active

His BMI was 26.

He was on diabetes medications (combination of glimepiride 1mg + metformin 500mg) twice day. His HBA1c was 7.8

He was very disciplined in his exercise and diet.

He used to play golf on weekends.

He could manage his stress levels.

I counselled him on fasting and low carbohydrates diet.

I gradually reduced his medication to simple metformin 500 twice a day.

He was enthusiastic to follow fasting.

He followed his fasting 16 hrs a day – 6 days a week.

After 3 months, his HBA1c reduced to 6.5%.

He felt good with low carbohydrates and fasting protocol.

I stopped his diabetes medications advised him to follow 16 hrs fasting 4 to 5 days week and 24 hrs fast once a week.

Over the next couple of months, his HBA1c reduced to 6.3% without medications.

Later he attended my wellness workshop too. Since last one year he is on a diabetes reversal mode with lifestyle changes as described above.

Case 4

Pradeep. Aged 36 years
Young IT engineer who was referred to me by one of my friends.
He used to have typical South Indian diet with predominantly more of carbohydrates.
He takes beer with oily foods twice a week.
He has put on weight of 10 kgs in the last one year.
His present weight is 88 kgs and BMI is 31.

On his routine blood tests, he noticed his blood sugars were high.
He did FBS, PPBS and HBa1c.
All were high.
His FBS: 200, PPBS: 350 and HBA1c 8.5

He was in shock after seeing his reports.
He couldn't believe he is now diabetic.

I counselled him to follow healthy lifestyle consistently with grain free diet, exercise, intermittent fasting and meditation.

I didn't start him on any medications in his first visit.

After 4 weeks his FBS came down to 140 and PPBS came down to 210.

He also lost 3 kg weight.

He became confident to follow low carbohydrate diet and fasting.

After next 2 months, his HBa1c reduced to 6.8 and fasting/after food sugars became normal. His weight reduced by 8 kgs.

He started feeling good and active. Over another month, his HBA1c reduced to 6.4.

Now he is used to following the lifestyle and diet which reversed his diabetes status.

Though he faced difficulties initially in changing diet habits, he gradually got used to it and won over diabetes.

References

1. Art and science of low carbohydrates living: Jeff S. Volek, Ph.D, RD Stephen D. Phinney, MD, Ph.D

2. Franz, MJ. The history of diabetes nutrition therapy. Diabetes Voice. 2004 Dec; 49: 30–33.

3. World Health Organization. Global report on diabetes. 2016.

4. Weiss R, Dufour S, et al. Pre-diabetes in obese youth: a syndrome of impaired glucose tolerance, severe insulin resistance, and altered myocellular and abdominal fat partitioning. Lancet. 2003; 362(9388): 951–957.

5. Reversing type 2 diabetes starts with ignoring the guidelines. TEDxPerdueU. https://www.youtube.com/watch?v=da1vvigy5tQ. Accessed 2017 Jun 14.

6. Rubino F. Medical research: Time to think differently about diabetes. Nature. 2016 May 24. Available from: http://www.nature.com/news/medical-research-time-to-think-differently-about-diabetes-1.19955. Accessed 2017 Jun 6.

7. Hughes T, Davies M. Thousands of diabetics adopt high-protein low-carb diet in backlash against official NHS eating plan. The Daily Mail. 2016 May 31. http://www.dailymail.co.uk/news/article-3617076/Diabetes-patients-defy-NHS-Thousands-rebel-against-guidelines-controlling-condition-diet-low-carbohydrates.html. Accessed 2017 Jun 12.

8. Jackson I, et al. Effect of fasting on glucose and insulin metabolism of obese patients. Lancet. 1969; 293(7589): 285–287.

9. Wareham NJ. The long-term benefits of lifestyle interventions for prevention of diabetes. Lancet Diabetes & Endocrinology. 2014 Jun; 2(6): 441–442.

10. Ramachandran A, et al. The Indian Diabetes Prevention Programme shows that lifestyle modification and metformin prevent type 2 diabetes in Asian Indian subjects with impaired glucose tolerance (IDP-1). Diabetologia. 2006; 49(2): 289–297.

11. Fung, Jason. "Intensive Dietary Management." Available from: www.IDMprogram.com

Good Reads – Suggestion

1. Periodic fasting by Jason fung

2. Pioppy diet by Dr. Aseem Malhotra

3. Diabetes – code by Dr.jason fung

4. Your diabetic questions answered by Jenny rahl

5. Blood sugar solution – Dr. Mark Hyman

6. Ancient wisdom for modern health – Mark, Bunn

7. Low Carb, High Fat food revolution – DR. ANDREAS EENFELDT